I0489056

CAREERS IN
EPIDEMIOLOGY
PUBLIC HEALTH PROFESSIONALS

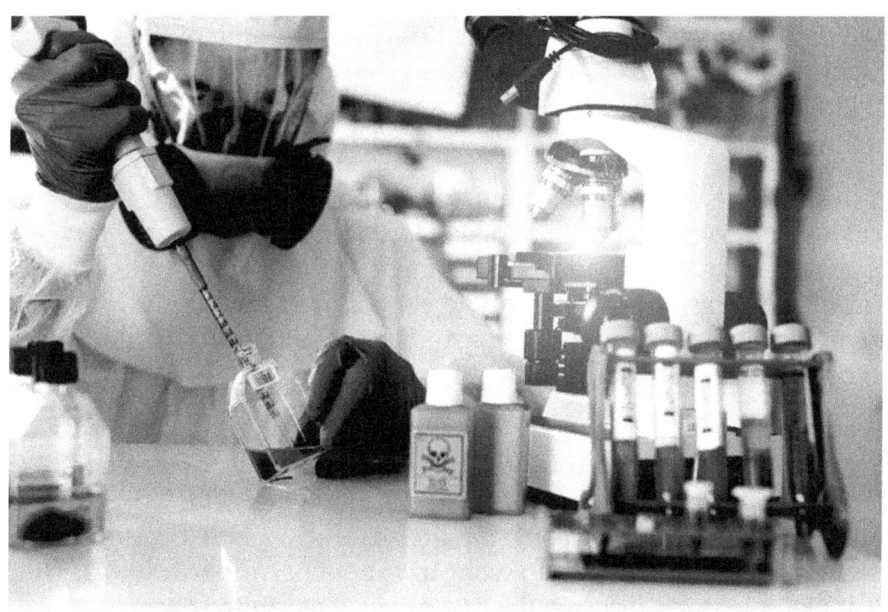

EPIDEMIOLOGISTS ARE SCIENTISTS who study diseases and other health risks within specific populations, such as geographical areas, cultures, occupations, demographic groups, or those who are genetically connected. They are "disease detectives," so-called because they are the investigators who discover how and where disease outbreaks start, then find ways to prevent them from spreading and recurring in the future.

It is believed that the first epidemiologist was Hippocrates, who studied how the outbreaks of different diseases correlated with environmental factors in Ancient Greece. That was nearly 2500 years ago. Since then, epidemiologists have saved millions of lives. They prevented the return of the Black Plague, identified how AIDS was transmitted, and quickly put a stop to the recent outbreak of Ebola in the US. These are just a few historical examples. The types of diseases that epidemiologists study are vast, ranging from food poisoning, to "clusters" of children with cancer, to mad cow disease.

The work of epidemiologists is based on intense research, which involves the collection of samples and data, and the application of statistical analysis. Much of it is accomplished in laboratories, but many of these professionals never set foot in a lab. Instead, they might be found in hospitals informing the medical staff of infectious outbreaks, or developing containment solutions for infections within the facility. Some work for pharmaceutical companies working on new drugs or monitoring vaccine development. Others may be out in epidemic ravaged communities, ensuring public safety as quarantine officers or investigating possible toxic agents in the environment. Still others are employed in the academic world, teaching and conducting research at universities.

To do this work, epidemiologists must be good with numbers, particularly statistics, in order to collect and accurately analyze data. That skill is of primary importance, but there is plenty more to learn before entering this career. You should expect to spend about six years following high school acquiring a master's degree in public health (MPH) or a related field, such as health, biology, medicine, or statistics.

When exploring an epidemiology career, you will find plenty of attractive features. For example, you will be generously compensated for your contribution to the public health of the world. The working conditions are generally excellent, the hours rarely include overtime, and travel is an option for those who want to experience other cultures. The future looks bright for future epidemiologists. The United States is placing a high priority on building up the nation's public health workforce. There are many questions that bright, energetic people are needed to help answer. What does this mean for you? It means that with a degree in public health, you will enjoy unparalleled job security and a career path filled with advancement opportunities. Best of all, you will be working in an exciting field that offers the personal and professional satisfaction of saving countless lives.

WHAT YOU CAN DO NOW

THERE ARE MULTIPLE PATHS TO becoming an epidemiologist, but all require a high level of education. Prepare yourself by getting a good academic foundation during your high school years. Take advantage of all the advanced level math courses and science courses that are offered. If a statistics course is available, take it. Enroll in courses that will help you hone your written and oral communications skills, and become computer savvy. Foreign language can also be very useful since it is common for epidemiologists to collaborate with people from around the world. Stay focused and make yourself a competitive candidate for the college of your choice. Aim for a GPA of 3.0 at a minimum – higher if you can.

Contact organizations like the Area Health Education Center to find health career fairs and ask about other opportunities for career exploration. Consider participating in the epidemiology competition through Health Occupations Students of America (HOSA). Subscribe to Vital Signs, a web publication of the Centers for Disease Control and Prevention (CDC). Do your research to discover how many areas of people's lives are affected by epidemiological data – and how many ways you can get involved.

Talk to epidemiologists in your community. If you live in a small town or rural area, you may have to travel to the nearest city. Contact research hospitals and universities and ask for assistance making connections. Speak with as many different professionals as you can. Their advice is invaluable. Each one of them will have different stories to tell you about epidemiology in general and their work in particular. Be sure to ask what they like and do not like about the career, what their average workday looks like, and where they went to school. Try to arrange to job shadow at least one epidemiologist to see what a working day in the field is really like.

Get a head start on your education with some free online courses in public health. The Council on Education for Public Health (CEPH) website includes a list of more than 200 free courses, many from top universities.

HISTORY OF THE PROFESSION

THE ORIGINS OF EPIDEMIOLOGY CAN BE traced back nearly 2500 years to Ancient Greece. In fact, the term "epidemiology" is derived from Greek, meaning "the study of what is upon the people." Most people recognize the Greek physician Hippocrates as the "father of medicine." Few realize he was also the first epidemiologist. It had always been believed that the source of disease was supernatural in nature. Hippocrates wrote in his essay, *On Airs, Waters, and Places,* that there was a much more logical cause for sickness. He was the first to link environmental and behavioral factors with the occurrence of disease, particularly when it was widespread.

In 1543, Italian physician Girolamo Fracastoro, wrote *De Contagione et Contagiosis Morbis* (translation: Of Contagions and Contagious Diseases). In the book, he set forth the theory – radical at that time – that the cause of disease was particles so small, they were invisible to the naked eye. He asserted that the particles were spread by air, multiplied spontaneously, and could be destroyed by fire. He also suggested that personal and environmental hygiene could prevent disease from starting or spreading. Fracastoro's "germ theory" received little support from the medical and scientific community since there was no physical evidence to provide proof. It would be 300 years before Fracastoro's theory became irrefutable, thanks to the work of Louis Pasteur and Robert Koch.

Not all early epidemiologists were physicians. An important contributor to the field was a merchant of men's clothing and amateur statistician named John Graunt. In his book, *Natural and Political Observations Made Upon the Bills of Mortality,* Graunt analyzed the mortality rolls of early modern London at the onset of the Great Plague. He was the first to be able to statistically quantify patterns of birth, death, disease occurrence, and disparities between various demographic groups and environments. The landmark publication provided, for the first time, statistical evidence supporting numerous theories on disease, as well as dispelling as many erroneous ideas. The book was first published in 1662 and by 1676, there were five editions.

In the early 1800s, William Farr built upon Graunt's work by collecting and analyzing Britain's vital statistics. He collected and evaluated those data and reported his findings to health authorities. Farr developed many of the methods used today in vital statistics and disease classification. He is widely recognized as the father of modern vital statistics and surveillance.

One of the most famous epidemiologists in history was anesthesiologist John Snow, another London resident. A contemporary of William Farr, Snow is considered one of the fathers of modern epidemiology due to his investigations into the cause of a cholera epidemic in Soho, London, in 1854. It was 20 years before the microscope was invented, yet Snow was able to discover not only the cause of the disease, but also how to prevent its recurrence. Ending the cholera outbreak was rightfully considered a major event in the history of public health. Snow not only stopped a deadly epidemic, he was able to establish a course of action to investigate outbreaks of disease that is still used today. With few exceptions, his research and recommendations for prevention were not put into practice until after his death. It was not until the latter part of the 1800s that investigators of disease outbreaks began to utilize epidemiological methods.

Prior to the 20th century, investigators were primarily concerned with acute infectious diseases. In the 1930s and 1940s, epidemiologists extended their methods to noninfectious diseases. Since World War II, epidemiology has been applied to the entire range of health-related conditions, behaviors, and attitudes. For example, the work of two British epidemiologists in the 1950s led to groundbreaking research that linked smoking to lung cancer. William Doll and Austin Bradford Hill are responsible for turning the subject of epidemiology into a rigorous science based on very strong statistical support. They also pioneered the randomized clinical trials that have been used ever since to research chronic disease.

One of the most far-reaching applications of epidemiology occurred in the 1960s and early 1970s. Health workers used epidemiologic methods to eradicate naturally occurring smallpox worldwide. It was an achievement of epic proportions.

In the 1980s, epidemiology extended beyond disease to include studies of injuries and violence. A decade later, the field was expanded yet again to include the related fields of molecular and genetic epidemiology. However, despite exciting new arenas for epidemiologists to practice, infectious diseases have remained the number one subject of concern. New infectious agents challenged epidemiologists who had never before encountered the likes of Ebola virus, Human Immunodeficiency Virus (HIV), Acquired Immunodeficiency Syndrome (AIDS), Legionella, and Severe Acute Respiratory Syndrome (SARS). Epidemiologists also did not expect diseases such as Mycobacterium tuberculosis and Avian influenza to become drug-resistant after previously being treated successfully.

Since the 1990s, epidemiology has no longer been concerned solely with natural transmission of infectious organisms. Rather, epidemiologists now have to be prepared to deal with the deliberate spread of disease through biological warfare and bioterrorism.

In the late 20th century, with advances in the biomedical sciences, new specialties have been introduced to the rapidly expanding scope of epidemiology. Researchers specializing in molecular epidemiology are now able to examine and analyze disease at the molecular level. These professionals can examine the relationship between an exposure to a disease-causing agent and the resulting molecular pathologic signature of a disease such as cancer. This type of research has become increasingly common in recent years. Another specialty known as "genetic epidemiology" is being used to track genetic variations and disease. Genetic variation is typically determined using DNA from white blood cells. Genome-wide association studies (GWAS) are now routinely being performed to identify genetic risk factors for many diseases and health conditions.

Today, public health workers throughout the world accept and use epidemiology in their communities to solve day-to-day health problems of all kinds. The term epidemiology is no longer limited to the research of epidemic disease, but includes many non-disease, health conditions, such as high blood pressure and obesity.

WHERE YOU WILL WORK

THERE ARE ABOUT 6,000 EPIDEMIOLOGISTS at work in the United States. More than half work for federal, state, and local government agencies. One of the largest employers is the Centers for Disease Control and Prevention (CDC) in Atlanta, Georgia. It is not only the leading national public health institute in the US, but is also the largest organization of its kind in the world. It is best known for investigating virulent epidemics, but it actually comprises many different departments that deal with a variety of health issues such as occupational safety, vaccines, chronic diseases, and traveler protection. The second largest employer of epidemiologists in the US is the National Institutes of Health (NIH) in Bethesda, Maryland. The NIH is the primary federal agency responsible for biomedical and health-related research and is one of the world's preeminent medical research centers. Both of these employers are federal agencies of the US Department of Health and Human Services. At the state and local levels, government-employed epidemiologists typically work in public health departments, hospitals, and schools.

Many epidemiologists work at colleges and universities, conducting research and teaching. Some are employed by for-profit pharmaceutical companies, private life science research and development facilities, health insurance companies, hospitals, and medical device manufacturers. Jobs within these organizations cover a wide range, such as technical consulting, research, clinical development, and market research.

Epidemiologists can also work in nonprofit organizations. These employers are usually organizations dealing directly with public health issues. Those employed by nonprofits often do public health advocacy work. Epidemiologists involved in research are rarely advocates, however, because scientific research is expected to be unbiased.

Work Environment

The typical epidemiologist works in a clean, well-lit office and/or laboratory. In the office, an epidemiologist will spend time at the computer, studying data and writing or reading reports. In the laboratory, the work is more technical, focusing on research and testing. Although epidemiology can involve dangerous chemicals or pathogens, there is little risk for laboratory workers because they are well trained and take extensive safety precautions.

Work environments can vary widely, however, especially for those who work in the field. Those who work for state and local public health departments are typically involved in public outreach. They may need to travel to conduct surveys and clinical studies or support community education programs. Those working for federal agencies may be called upon to support emergency actions anywhere in the country.

Some specialists travel extensively. Infectious disease epidemiologists, for example, often travel beyond US borders to collect samples and conduct environmental investigations. This usually means traveling to developing countries and remote regions because in most cases, infectious diseases have been greatly diminished in developed countries.

Work Schedules

Most epidemiologists work full time during normal business hours. However, hours are less predictable for those who have responsibilities during public health emergencies, who travel, or who work in developing countries. Fieldwork may also require occasional work on nights, weekends, or holidays.

THE WORK YOU WILL DO

EPIDEMIOLOGISTS INVESTIGATE AND ANALYZE the causes and spreading of disease, injury, and other health problems in human populations. Whether it is food poisoning affecting consumers in multiple states or the initial discovery of mad cow disease, these are the professionals that are asked to determine the source of the outbreak, what the risks are, who is at risk, and how to prevent further incidences. They accomplish this through specific types of statistical analysis that reveals patterns within targeted population groups.

Their work does not necessarily involve epidemics, but it often does. Whether it is a particularly bad season for the flu or an unusual number of children in a small town who have succumbed to cancer, epidemiologists seek to find ways to reduce such negative health incidences through research, community education, and public health policy.

Even though humans are living longer and many diseases are no longer the imminent threat they once were, epidemiologists remain vigilant protectors of our collective health. New disease outbreaks, such as Ebola, Salmonella, and the Zika virus, continue to pop up unexpectedly with tragic results. Diseases that were previously considered extinct, such as measles, scarlet fever, whooping cough, and tuberculosis, sometimes make a comeback. In either case, it is up to epidemiologists to device ways to put an end to the problem.

Research Epidemiologists

Epidemiologists are classified into two groups: research and clinical. Research epidemiologists conduct research in order to understand, eradicate, and control infectious diseases. They study health problems that affect the entire body, such as AIDS or any of the common autoimmune diseases. They may also focus only on localized infections, such as those of the digestive tract, lung, or brain.

Epidemiology research generally involves gathering medical and health information from the field or historical data, analyzing the data collected, and presenting the findings. The goal is to determine how diseases originate, how they spread, and perhaps most importantly, how they can be treated or eradicated. The findings are often used to develop or change public health initiatives.

In addition to studying the origin and spread of contagious life-threatening diseases, research epidemiologists analyze medical conditions that occur as a result of generalized exposure, such as foodborne illnesses, water or air pollution, or lead poisoning. They also research the trends within populations of survivors of certain diseases, such as cancer, in order to determine what has been proven to be the most effective treatments. That is very useful information that can be disseminated across the entire population.

Clinical Epidemiologists

Clinical epidemiologists also conduct research, but their work is not restricted to the laboratory. In addition to working in an office or laboratory, they are often in the field meeting with doctors and others involved with public health issues. They may be enlisted as consultants at hospitals, informing the medical staff of infectious outbreaks and suggesting containment solutions. Unlike research epidemiologists who tend to work behind the scenes, clinical epidemiology is often patient oriented. For that reason, they may also be trained as medical doctors or in an allied healthcare field.

Clinical epidemiologists are often called upon to conduct research on sudden disease outbreaks. In this case, they have to work quickly, while making sure the analytical measures and data interpretations are accurate. They use their findings to develop complex disease control procedures and help public health departments fine tune response protocols. Clinical epidemiologists are also tasked with developing procedures and policies regarding disease control for hospitals, nursing homes, and schools.

Job Tasks

The specific day-to-day job duties of an epidemiologist will vary depending on the employer and level of experience. Regardless of where they work, there are basic tasks that apply to most epidemiologists. Here are some things that a general epidemiologist with fewer than five years of experience might do during a typical workday:

- Participate in research on a specific disease or adverse health condition.

- Collect data through observations, interviews, surveys, and sampling of blood and other bodily fluids.

- Analyze data using statistical models in order to determine the cause of the health problem being researched.

- Review current scientific literature.

- Study historical and contemporary population lifestyle characteristics to isolate influencing factors such as pollution, misinformation, alcohol and drug abuse, poor hygiene, or lack of healthy foods.

- Use computer-modeling software to judge the potential impact of disease and health changes within a specific population.

- Write the reports for a complete research project.

- Participate in community outreach programs by teaching the public and their leaders how to protect their health.

More experienced epidemiologists are given greater responsibilities. Their daily routines might include the following:

- Design and manage large-scale interdisciplinary projects on public health problems to find ways to prevent and treat them.

- Support strategic initiatives by writing, speaking, or advocating for changes regarding a certain public health issue as new research warrants.

- Manage public health programs by planning a variety of educational activities.

- Produce detailed technical documents that will be used for proposals, presentations, bidding for projects, and soliciting government or private funding.

- Monitor regulatory healthcare policies and make recommendations for changes.

- Present findings from important research or public health programs to community leaders, government policymakers, health practitioners, and senior management of private organizations.

- Supervise professional, technical, and clerical personnel.

- Develop and improve research methodology.

Specialty Areas

Epidemiology is a diverse field that is expanding into new areas all the time. It is becoming increasingly common for professionals in the field to specialize in one or more areas. Some of the most popular specialties include infection control, pharmaceuticals, disaster and emergency response, environmental health, and molecular epidemiology.

Infection control epidemiologists deal with public health problems within hospitals and medical facilities.

It has been widely publicized that lives are lost because of the spread of infections such as MRSA within hospitals. Infection control epidemiologists are responsible for preventing the spread of infections within their facilities. In addition to enforcing hygiene procedures, their daily tasks generally include collecting and analyzing health data within the hospital. Specifically, they record observations, conduct surveys and interviews, take blood samples, and collect other bodily samples.

Pharmaceutical epidemiologists study how various drugs affect the health and physiology of a particular human population.

They do research and conduct clinical studies of drugs and procedures while monitoring side effects and results. They also study how social trends and habits could spread certain diseases. The goal of this work is to find new, more effective and safer treatments and medications for a variety of health problems. Much of the work is conducted in the laboratory, testing how different combinations and amounts of chemicals react with tissue samples.

Disaster and emergency response is an exciting specialty, and ideal for those who want to get out of the laboratory and do some hands-on work. These professionals are the ones made famous by movies like *Outbreak*. Disaster epidemiologists spend the bulk of their time in the office and/or laboratory, studying the factors that might lead to disasters and finding ways to reduce adverse results. The work involves using advanced epidemiologic methods, such as surveillance systems, to identify injuries and diseases that may be caused by the disaster. These professionals often interact with people in the general population, educating community leaders and helping develop public health preparedness procedures. They are also responsible for informing relief workers of all possible dangers in certain situations.

Environmental health epidemiologists study the health effects of exposure to environmental contaminants such as air pollution, hazardous waste, radiation, heavy metals, pesticides, and asbestos.

Adverse effects of these hazards may vary widely, from developmental delays in children to neurological disorders and cardiopulmonary diseases in adults. These professionals also investigate unknown causes of "clusters," such as high incidences of cancer or autism in a particular community. Environmental epidemiologists are often called upon to advise government agencies on acceptable levels of exposure. This is vital work that has helped protect the public from the harmful effects of mercury in fish, mold exposure, and high ozone days.

Molecular epidemiology involves the application of molecular biology to the study of public health.

The goal of this work is to determine what genetic and environmental risk factors, identified at the molecular level, might contribute to the distribution of diseases within families and across general populations. Advanced techniques such as nucleic acid analysis allow epidemiologists to ascertain what causes diseases within a given population and to precisely measure exposures to a disease. Knowing this can potentially lead to disease prevention or the end of an outbreak.

Veterinary epidemiology involves diseases that are transmitted among animals and between animals and humans.

This is a critical job considering the prevalence of animal-to-human transmission of infectious diseases, such as mad cow disease, avian influenza, and swine flu. The work is often time-sensitive, particularly when infectious diseases are emanating from grocery stores, restaurants, and meat production facilities with multi-state distribution. Many people can become ill or even die before the source is discovered.

Advancement

Epidemiology is an exciting field that is in serious need of experienced professionals. There are many opportunities for epidemiologists to advance their careers, either by moving laterally into a new specialty or moving up to management or consulting positions.

Becoming a supervisory epidemiologist is the first step into management. Depending on experience, the supervisory epidemiologist may be a team leader or a member of senior management. A team leader oversees a group of junior epidemiologists while managing one or more research projects. Senior managers may be a department head, heading up major research studies, or become involved in the organization's overall planning.

Some epidemiologists prefer the academic world. Anyone working for a university must become a faculty member and teach students. Some epidemiologists like teaching. Others will do it, but many because they are also given the opportunity to do cutting edge research in a noncompetitive environment. University sponsored research projects are typically conducted in world class laboratories complete with funding to cover the costs of any new equipment or travel expenses. Academic researchers often work on projects of critical importance. Their work often leads to major discoveries that influence the health of populations throughout the world, while impacting domestic policies related to public health.

STORIES OF EPIDEMIOLOGISTS AT WORK

I Practice Applied Epidemiology

"As an applied epidemiologist, I get to solve real problems in the real world. I started out conducting theoretical research studies, but I'm much happier being able to get out of the lab and seeing what my skills can do for people.

I have worked on a variety of projects, but currently my work involves monitoring and evaluating HIV programs in underdeveloped countries. The work requires that I spend about half my time traveling. I do get to interact directly with some of the people that may be affected by my work. I have always been interested in helping improve the health of underserved populations, whether they are in Mississippi or Cambodia. I could have chosen to become a doctor, but as an epidemiologist, I am able to impact entire communities simultaneously rather than one patient at a time.

Epidemiology allows me to combine my strong math skills with my interest in addressing social problems. I am constantly intrigued by the many different factors that contribute to the occurrences of diseases. It's like a big puzzle that I have to solve in order to help people lead healthier lives. Still, what I like best about my work is immersing myself in new cultures and working with people in other countries. It fascinates me how different our environments can be, yet we human beings are all very much alike. I can't think of another career that could be more intellectually and personally satisfying."

I Study the Causes of Cancer

"My employer is a major nonprofit organization devoted to finding a cure for cancer. My work currently focuses on research related to the high incidence of cancer in racial and ethnic minorities. In the future, however, I want to shift my attention to children. Most people don't realize that cancer is the leading cause of death by disease among children in the US. Although the cure rate has improved with greater chances of survival increased, the incidence of childhood cancer has been steadily increasing over the last few decades. I want to know why. Genetic mutations account for only a small percentage. I suspect there are environmental factors that could make childhood cancer highly preventable. I can't think of a more worthwhile subject for epidemiological research.

I had my doubts about pursuing a career in epidemiology. I assumed (wrongly) that my job would have me struck in front of a computer all day churning out faceless data when what I really wanted to do was help people. An internship quickly set me straight. My job is much more interactive than that. I regularly meet with collaborators from other organizations. I am often asked to give talks and meet with community representatives.

The best thing about my work is the way it constantly challenges me.

There is so much to learn! New discoveries are made every day in the field of cancer and yet with every answer, there are more questions.

If I had it to do over again, I would be more strategic in preparing for my career. I would set more challenging goals and ask for more help from mentors to achieve those goals. New epidemiologists should not underestimate the value of soliciting feedback. It's not that hard to find a senior researcher willing to be a mentor. If asked in the right way, people in this profession are very generous with their help.

Beyond that, my advice is to find and follow your passion. Epidemiology is a wonderfully diverse field with something of interest for everyone with the proper training. A public health degree can allow you to contribute to solutions to the many important issues facing our world. That includes how to prevent cancer as well as how to maintain optimal health if you have cancer."

PERSONAL QUALIFICATIONS

THE PRACTICE OF EPIDEMIOLOGY REQUIRES A VARIETY OF SKILLS, BUT PERHAPS THE SINGLE most important is the ability to understand and use statistics in a meaningful way. Any reasonably intelligent person can be trained to collect data. However, it is what is done with that data that matters. On the job, an epidemiologist must be able to draw credible conclusions from the data that can be applied to real world situations. Some epidemiologists are not directly involved in obtaining or analyzing data. Those professionals must still be able to assess the information, understand it, and test its accuracy and significance.

Other important skills needed to be successful in this career include:

Communications skills

Conducting fact-finding interviews is a big part of the epidemiologist's job. This requires listening carefully and paying great attention to detail. The ability to write clearly is necessary to work effectively with team members and other health professionals. Epidemiologists write many reports, opinion pieces, and original research papers. Members of the medical profession and community leaders look to these written documents for answers and recommendations they can understand.

When research leads to solid plans intended to prevent or solve a public health problem, those plans must be clear to everyone including the general public. It is one thing to explain statistics and patterns to healthcare workers. It is more difficult to describe a plan of action to ordinary citizens. Excellent speaking skills are necessary. Teaching skills are a big plus, especially for those involved in community outreach activities.

Passion for solving problems

Epidemiologists are confronted with the most challenging health problems facing the human population. It can be tedious and even frustrating at times. Having excellent problem solving skills are necessary for success in this career. To be fulfilled by the work, you must genuinely care about the lives you could be saving. Without feeling a deep connection to the health problem you are working to overcome, the work will eventually lose its appeal. Staying focused on the bigger picture will help you recognize the significance of the work you do every day.

Details and more details

Epidemiologists must be precise, both while gathering data and during analysis. They must be able to identify minute details and nuances in numerical data that even trained medical professionals would miss.

Math and technical skills

Advanced math and strong statistical skills are used in the design and administration of studies and surveys. While much of this work is accomplished with the aid of computer software, an epidemiologist must be proficient with such technical tools. During the first phase of data collection, the computer does the storage and much of the basic analysis. The epidemiologist must know how to view and process the information using data presentation software programs. Those who are successful in this field keep up with information technology advancements in data mining and predictive analytics.

ATTRACTIVE FEATURES

FOR ANY EPIDEMIOLOGIST, THE YEARS OF EDUCATION are long, but the time and effort spent are worth it. Right from the start, these professionals earn attractive salaries that easily cover all their needs. The reason most people pursue this career, however, is the opportunity to save lives on a huge scale. It is the type of work that is good for those who like to help people get better and live healthier lives. Epidemiologists enjoy the satisfaction that comes from investigating and solving problems related to disease. The problems are always serious and finding solutions is rarely easy. Those who enjoy intellectual challenges will thrive in this work.

Epidemiology offers a good amount of job flexibility. The field covers a broad spectrum, and the career can be taken in many different directions without returning to school for more training. There is a long list of job types and specialties to choose from. Some are perfect for those who like pure research and prefer to work in a laboratory. Others involve interaction with people, such as patients, doctors, community and business leaders, government policymakers, professionals from other disciplines, and people in other countries. Travel is also a possibility for those who want to see the world and learn about other cultures.

Those who do continue their education will find even more doors open to them. A PhD or medical degree allows an epidemiologist to go into high-level research in large facilities or universities. They can also join university faculties or advance to more managerial positions.

UNATTRACTIVE ASPECTS

TO BECOME AN EPIDEMIOLOGIST, you will have to work hard, study many hours, and master an enormous amount of information. This job requires extensive knowledge since there are several academic studies involved in the work. The work itself can also be very intense. Trying to put an end to an epidemic affecting thousands of people presents an awesome responsibility. The work can also be depressing. Focuses on disease and suffering are not for everyone, although most epidemiologists rate the stress level as only moderate.

There are elements of risk in this job. Some of the diseases you will study are lethal. There are viruses that can make you very sick and even kill you. For that reason, epidemiologists receive a great deal of training in safety procedures. Those who heed the required precautions are rarely harmed.

Containing or preventing a disease often comes down to changing human behavior. It can be as simple as the need for routine handwashing. Yet getting people to change their habits can be the toughest part of this job. It takes patience and good communications skills to explain why certain practices are necessary and address any misconceptions. Trying to convince patients to engage in safe practices may not be easy, but doing so can ultimately be rewarding.

Epidemiology is not known for being fast paced. It is often a slow moving process that can go on for years. During that time, the daily grind may become mundane or even tedious. There will certainly be times when daily tasks will seem dull. To avoid boredom, successful epidemiologists keep their eyes on the prize – the eradication of potentially deadly diseases. There are also ample opportunities for travel, or to specialize in another type of work that may be more interesting.

EDUCATION AND TRAINING

EPIDEMIOLOGISTS NEED AT LEAST A MASTER'S DEGREE from an accredited college or university. This is usually the Master of Public Health (MPH), but it may be called Master of Science in Public Health (MSPH), or Master of Medical Science in Public Health (MMSPH). Another possibility is a master's degree in health sciences, biology, or statistics. Those who are interested in working with the public health initiative are advised to consider pursuing a degree in sociology. There are very few universities that offer epidemiology majors at the undergraduate level. You need to graduate from college before you embark on your professional training.

Regardless of your major, as an undergraduate you should include classes in public health, biology, chemistry, statistics, and other related subjects. Some graduate schools require an undergraduate degree in a certain major. Be sure to check with your guidance counselor before making a final decision about your major.

There are hundreds of Schools of Public Health in the US. The Association of Schools and Programs of Public Health (ASPPH) accredit many. Just as many are accredited by the Council on Education for Public Health (CEPH). Most are campus-based, but CEPH has also accredited a small number of MPH online programs. Some of the best Schools of Public Health in the United States are:

Johns Hopkins University in Baltimore

University of North Carolina in Chapel Hill

Harvard University

University of Michigan in Ann Arbor

Columbia University

You should start to apply to Schools of Public Health when you are a senior in college. To improve the chances of admission to the school of your choice, try to get some work experience while you are an undergraduate. You can do this by interning in epidemiological research facilities or medical labs. Be sure to solicit letters of recommendations from any working epidemiologists you meet during those experiences.

A master's degree program in public health will provide a broad overview of public health topics. Initial courses will include math and biostatistics, behavioral studies, biological and physical sciences, health services research and administration, immunology, and toxicology, and other public health subjects. You will learn everything from how to handle dangerous viruses in the lab to how to organize a public health initiative. Advanced courses will prepare you to apply your knowledge in the workplace. Those classes will emphasize survey design, statistical methodology, medical informatics, multiple regression, and practical applications of data. You will review previous biomedical research and compare various healthcare systems.

Many master's degree programs in public health require students to participate in an internship that may take up to a year to complete.

Education for Career Advancement

Most epidemiologists have a master's degree in public health with an emphasis in epidemiology. There are some epidemiologists who also go on to earn a doctorate degree (Doctor of Philosophy). With a PhD, an epidemiologist can work in larger facilities, direct major research projects, become a full professor at a university, and generally be qualified to take on positions with greater responsibility at a higher level of pay. It takes a minimum of four years of full-time study to earn a PhD as an epidemiologist. Some programs allow you to earn an MPH and a PhD together, which saves some time.

Some epidemiologists are also physicians. These are usually people who want to work in clinical epidemiology. A medical degree allows an epidemiologist to administer drugs to patients during clinical research studies and trials.

Certification

The Certification Board of Infection Control and Epidemiology (CBIC) provides voluntary certification for epidemiologists who have worked within the infection control industry for at least two years. To be awarded the Certified Infection Control (CIC) certificate, applicants must have a post-secondary degree and pass an exam. The certificate is good for five years. After that, recertification is accomplished by passing the Self Achievement Recertification Examination (SARE). The CIC certificate represents competence in the actual practice of infection prevention and control and healthcare epidemiology. It is not intended for new graduates, but for those who are actively accountable for the infection prevention and control program within their current positions.

Experienced epidemiologists can advance their careers with continuing education and additional certification programs offered by the Association for Professionals in Infection Control and Epidemiology (APIC).

EARNINGS

ACCORDING TO THE MOST RECENT INFORMATION, epidemiologists earn a median annual income of just under $70,000. New graduates are offered starting salaries around $45,000 on average, and many of these professionals will go on to reach more than $115,000 in annual earnings. Whether an epidemiologist ultimately achieves compensation at the highest level depends on the number of years of experience, qualifications and certifications, geographic location, and the type of industry.

Salaries are often based on the years of experience in the field. According to some surveys, an epidemiologist with at least 15 years of experience will earn about 10 percent more than the national median.

At the other end of the spectrum, a beginner with less than one year on the job will earn about 10 percent less than the national median.

Geography plays a big factor in determining salaries. Professionals working in a large city, an esteemed university, or major research hospital are at a distinct advantage. Simply living in the right place pays off. Above average yearly salaries are enjoyed by those living in the following metropolitan areas:

San Diego	$114,000
Denver	$111,000
Durham	$105,000
Oakland	$103,000
Boston	$102,000
San Francisco	$102,000

Type of industry also has an impact on what an epidemiologist's salary might be. Industries that pay especially well include pharmaceutical manufacturing, scientific research and consulting, and computer systems design. Those working in scientific research, for example, earn more than $110,000 a year on average.

The median annual wages for epidemiologists among the biggest types of employers are as follows:

- Research and development in the physical, engineering, and life sciences
  $92,000

- Private medical and surgical hospitals
  $78,000

- Colleges, universities, and professional schools (both private and public)
  $68,000

- State government agencies
  $65,000

- Local government agencies
  $63,000

Although a large percentage of epidemiologists work for state or local government agencies, that is not where earnings are the highest. Professionals in government employment earn about $65,000, which is below the national median. Their non-government colleagues, however, generally make above the national median, between $80,000 and $110,000. Those not directly employed by a government agency are often the beneficiaries of government funding though. This is particularly true for research epidemiologists who work on large, important projects.

In addition to a base salary, there are typically good benefits. Benefits for epidemiologists tend to be generous, in part because so many work in the public sector. Exactly what benefits might be provided vary by employer, but most packages include holiday pay, vacation days, sick days, retirement plans such as a 401K, paid personal days, profit sharing, bonuses, etc. Medical benefits are almost always included and dental coverage is quite common.

OPPORTUNITIES

EMPLOYMENT GROWTH WILL BE about equal to the average growth for all occupations, over the coming decade. The number of new epidemiology jobs will be less than 1,000 since the field is so small to begin with. The unemployment rate is a more revealing statistic. The national unemployment rate of epidemiologists is a tiny fraction, probably close to zero. Even the unemployment rate of all health services professionals is greater. It is clear that the work of epidemiologists is important and necessary. The relatively small number of job openings should not put off those individuals who are considering following this career path. Once trained, a new epidemiologist can expect to find a good position with exceptional job security.

The concentration of epidemiologist jobs in state and local government agencies is expected to continue. Demand will be strong over the next 10 years, but job growth is no greater than that of most other occupations. The problem is primarily budgetary. Job growth in this arena revolves around the fiscal health of the state or local government. Unlike private organizations and the federal government, local and state governments have to follow the dictates of budgetary limitations. In some cases, state and local agencies put strict austerity measures in place that put a serious damper on hiring. At the same time, however, government regulations have increased the need for epidemiologists in hospitals, both private and public. More than ever, hospitals are expected to track health outcomes and address local population health concerns – something only epidemiologists are trained to do.

The healthcare industry is booming and medical recordkeeping technologies have been developed to keep up with it all. With continued improvements in information technologies, epidemiologists will be able to analyze medical information on a level not previously possible. One especially helpful technology is Big Data, which allows extremely large data sets to be computationally analyzed to reveal patterns, trends, and associations, especially relating to human behavior and interactions. Although developed for big business, Big Data is well suited for epidemiology. Continuing statistical and mapping software will also help epidemiologists track health outcomes and demographic data with more accuracy than ever. These technological developments require the expertise of epidemiologists to be of any value.

Interest in public health and epidemiology has increased dramatically over the past decade. The number of graduates pursuing careers in epidemiology has likewise grown, creating some strong competition for the top jobs. However, applicants will find that the toughest jobs to get are not necessarily the best. There is more competition for general, some would say routine, research than for more interesting specialties. Because epidemiology is a diverse field, opportunities can easily be found if one takes a broad view. Those who are willing to work in any of the various specialty areas rarely have trouble finding work.

GETTING STARTED

AS A NEW GRADUATE, YOUR RÉSUMÉ may be a bit spotty. There are several ways you can engage in a successful job search. The first involves networking. The epidemiology community is relatively small, making it an ideal environment for networking. This is an activity you should start while still in school. There are numerous ways you can build connections. First, talk to your professors during office hours and at social events. Professors can also be extremely valuable. They can serve as references for your job applications and recommend the best professional conferences and talks for you to attend. Showing your face at epidemiology or public health events will help demonstrate your dedication to the field. Professors usually know professional epidemiologists working in the field. That means they can provide networking contacts to get you a job interview or an informal job recommendation. Direct connections like that can help you land a job before anyone else hears about it.

Join organizations at your school that focus on the type of work you are interested in. There may not be an epidemiology club, but there might be a malaria awareness group, for example. Actively participate and consider taking a leadership position. Being part of a group like that will help develop your communication skills and will bring you many new connections.

Joining professional epidemiological organizations can provide valuable opportunities to both network and gather additional experience. There are dozens of suitable organizations to choose from. Each offers exposure to what different types of epidemiologists do as well as provide opportunities to gain more experience – something your résumé could use! For example, the Association for Professionals in Infection Control actively solicits volunteers. The Center of Disease Control and Prevention has four training and fellowship programs for epidemiology students and graduates:

- The Epidemiology Elective Program
- The CDC Experience Applied Epidemiology Fellowship
- The Epidemic Intelligence Service
- The CDC/CSTE Applied Epidemiology Fellowship Program

Beyond networking and training programs, there are other ways to find job opportunities. Read through medical journals. Most have "help wanted" sections. Also, look on the websites of national health service organizations. Employment agencies can be useful, especially those that specialize in the healthcare industry. Look for those that focus on closely related fields, such as medical research careers. One of the best ways to research the job market is to consult with the career services office at your school. Your school's placement center should have job listings.

Before any job interview, make sure that your résumé is polished. Be prepared to speak confidently. You will need to discuss in detail your previous research experience (school-related research counts) as well as your interests for the future. Hiring is usually done by a hiring committee. Every member of that committee will want to know what makes you a special candidate. Be able to answer that question.

ASSOCIATIONS

■ **National Institutes of Health (NIH)**
http://www.nih.gov

■ **American Public Health Association (APHA)**
http://www.apha.org

■ **Society for Healthcare Epidemiology of America (SHEA)**
http://www.shea-online.org

■ **The American College of Epidemiology (ACE)**
http://acepidemiology.org

■ **The Association for Professionals in Infection Control and Epidemiology (APIC)**
http://www.apic.org

■ **The American Epidemiological Society (AES)**
http://americanepidemiologicalsociety.org

■ **The Certification Board of Infection Control and Epidemiology (CBIC)**
https://www.cbic.org

■ **Health Occupations Students of America (HOSA)**
http://www.hosa.org

■ **The National Area Health Education Center Organization**
http://www.nationalahec.org

■ **Council on Education for Public Health (CEPH)**
http://ceph.org/accredited

■ **Association of Schools and Programs of Public Health (ASPPH)** http://www.aspph.org

■ **Public Health Foundation (PHF)**
http://www.phf.org

PUBLICATION

■ Vital Signs
http://www.cdc.gov/vitalsigns

WEBSITES

■ The Epidemiology Elective Program
http://www.cdc.gov/epielective

■ The CDC Experience Applied Epidemiology Fellowship
http://www.cdc.gov/cdcexperiencefellowship

■ The Epidemic Intelligence Service http://www.cdc.gov/eis

■ The CDC/CSTE Applied Epidemiology Fellowship Program
http://www.cste.org/?page=Fellowship

■ Center for Disease Control and Prevention (CDC) Job Board
https://jobs.cdc.gov

Copyright 2017
Institute For Career Research
CAREERS INTERNET DATABASE

www.careers-internet.org

www.ingramcontent.com/pod-product-compliance
Lightning Source LLC
Chambersburg PA
CBHW061239180526
45170CB00003B/1372